Preventing Tinnitus

Lifestyle Changes And Habits

Dr, Tiffany J. Bozeman

CONTENT

CHAPTER ONE

Tinnitus: An Overview

Millions of individuals throughout the globe suffer from tinnitus, which is a common ailment. It is distinguished by the ability to perceive sound without an external input. This noise may seem like a roaring sound, ringing, buzzing, or even hissing. The sound may be present in one or both ears, it may be constant or sporadic. A person's quality of life may be substantially impacted by a chronic illness like tinnitus.

The many facets of tinnitus, including what it is, its causes, forms, and symptoms, will be covered in this chapter.

What exactly is tinnitus

The sense of sound without an external trigger is known as tinnitus. It is a sign of an underlying issue rather than a sickness. One or both ears may hear the sound, which might vary in volume, pitch, and frequency. Both subjective and objective tinnitus exist. The most typical sort of tinnitus, subjective, can only be heard by the person who has it. On the other hand, objective tinnitus is audible to both the sick person and others around them. It is brought on by the body's physical noises, such as blood flow turbulence or muscular spasms.

The Root Causes Of Tinnitus

TNumerous factors may lead to tinnitus, including:

1. Hearing loss: Tinnitus and hearing loss, particularly age-related hearing loss, are often linked. Tinnitus may be brought on by damaged sensory cells in the inner ear, which can mistakenly communicate with the brain.

2. Loud noise exposure: Loud noise exposure, particularly prolonged exposure, might result in tinnitus. People who often go to loud music events or work in noisy workplaces may experience this.

3. Ear infections and injuries: Tinnitus may be brought on by ear infections or trauma. This is due to the possibility that they may harm the auditory nerve or the inner ear, which would cause the brain to receive inaccurate information.

4. Pharmaceuticals: Several pharmaceuticals, including aspirin,

NSAIDs, and some antibiotics, may result in tinnitus.

5. Medical Issues: Tinnitus may be brought on by disorders including Meniere's disease, excessive blood pressure, and thyroid issues.

Tinnitus Types

Tinnitus comes in two flavors: subjective and objective.

1. Subjective tinnitus: This sort of tinnitus, which is the most prevalent, can only be heard by the person who is experiencing it. It may be brought on by medical

disorders, hearing loss, exposure to loud noise, ear injuries or infections, medicines, or hearing loss.

2. Objective tinnitus is audible to both the afflicted person and others in the vicinity. It is brought on by the body's physical noises, such as blood flow turbulence or muscular spasms.

The Signs Of Tinnitus

Tinnitus symptoms might differ from person to person. The following are some of the most typical signs of tinnitus:

1. Ear noises such as ringing, buzzing, hissing, or roaring

2. A sporadic or constant sound

3. Hearing a sound in just one ear or both ears

4. Modifications in sound volume, pitch, and frequency

5. Hearing or concentration issues brought on by noise

6. Depression and anxiety because of how it affects the quality of life

Lifestyle Modifications to Prevent Tinnitus

A person's quality of life may be greatly impacted by tinnitus. Tinnitus does not yet have a recognized treatment, but several lifestyle modifications may help avoid it or manage its symptoms. The many lifestyle modifications that people may undertake to avoid tinnitus will be covered in this chapter, including dietary adjustments, physical activity, stress management approaches, and sleep hygiene.

Dietary Modifications to Prevent Tinnitus

Diet has a significant impact on general health and well-being and may have an impact on tinnitus. Individuals may alter their diets in the following ways to avoid tinnitus:

1. Cutting down on salt: Eating a lot of salt may raise blood pressure, which can lead to tinnitus. Consuming less salt may assist those with high blood pressure to avoid developing tinnitus.

2. Steer clear of coffee and alcohol. These substances might disrupt ear blood flow, which can result in tinnitus. Tinnitus may be prevented by avoiding or consuming these things less often.

3. Eating foods high in antioxidants: By lowering oxidative stress in the body,

foods high in antioxidants, such as fruits and vegetables, may help prevent tinnitus.

4. Increasing magnesium intake: Magnesium is necessary for the auditory system to operate properly. Tinnitus may be avoided by increasing magnesium intake via diet or supplementation.

Tinnitus Prevention Through Exercise and Physical Activity

Tinnitus may be avoided with regular exercise and physical activity, among other health advantages. Exercise may help prevent tinnitus in several ways, including:

1. Increasing blood flow: Regular exercise may increase blood flow to the ears as well as the rest of the body. Tinnitus brought on by inadequate blood supply to the ear may be avoided in this way.

2. Reducing stress: Stress, which may cause tinnitus, can be reduced by exercise.

3. Enhancing general well-being: Exercise may enhance general well-being and lower the risk of illnesses that can lead to tinnitus.

Techniques for Reducing Stress to Prevent Tinnitus

Tinnitus may be significantly triggered by stress. Thus, lowering stress may aid in the prevention of tinnitus. Some methods for reducing the stress that people may employ to ward against tinnitus include:

1. Mindfulness and meditation may help decrease stress and improve relaxation, which can help avoid tinnitus.

2. Breathing exercises: By promoting relaxation and lowering stress levels,

breathing exercises may help prevent tinnitus.

3. Yoga: Yoga may prevent tinnitus by lowering stress and enhancing general well-being.

Tinnitus Prevention Through Good Sleep Practices

The habits and procedures people undertake to encourage restful sleep are referred to as sleep hygiene. Tinnitus may be triggered by poor sleep. As a result, maintaining proper sleep hygiene is crucial to avoiding tinnitus. To avoid tinnitus, people may follow several sleep hygiene practices, such as:

1. Making a regular sleep schedule: Maintaining a regular bedtime and wake-up time will enhance the body's circadian rhythm and improve the quality of your sleep.

2. Creating a tranquil sleeping environment: A peaceful, cozy, and dark sleeping environment may encourage high-quality sleep, which prevents tinnitus.

3. Avoiding coffee and alcohol before bedtime: These substances may interfere with sleep and cause tinnitus.

Tinnitus prevention may be significantly aided by changes in lifestyle. To avoid tinnitus, people may adjust their diets, engage in regular physical activity, learn stress management strategies, and practice excellent sleeping habits. Individuals may lower their chance of acquiring tinnitus or control its symptoms by implementing these lifestyle modifications.

CHAPTER TWO

Environmental Modifications to Prevent Tinnitus

In the onset and treatment of tinnitus, environmental variables may also have a big impact. We will discuss some of the environmental changes people can make to prevent tinnitus in this chapter, such as lowering noise exposure and protecting the ears in noisy environments, recognizing and avoiding workplace hazards that can cause tinnitus, setting up a secure home environment, and being mindful of noise exposure during travel and recreational activities.

Hearing Loss with Noise Exposure

Tinnitus is often brought on by loud noise exposure. Therefore, decreasing noise exposure is crucial for tinnitus prevention. Here are some strategies for lowering noise exposure:

1. Use hearing protection: Earmuffs or earplugs may help shield your ears from loud sounds.

2. Turn down the volume: Stay away from loud sounds, such as those made by

equipment, power tools, or loud music. Reduce the volume if you must be in a loud setting, or go away from the noisemaker.

3. Take rests: If you are subjected to loud noise for a long time, take pauses to give your hearing a rest.

Prevention of Tinnitus and Workplace Risks

Tinnitus may develop as a result of many job dangers, such as loud noise exposure, chemicals that are hazardous to the ears, and head trauma. The following are some methods to avoid occupational risks that might cause tinnitus:

1. Put on safety equipment. Depending on your line of work, you may need to put on respirators, earplugs, or helmets.

2. Be aware of your noise exposure: If your employment requires you to work in a loud setting, be aware of your exposure to noise and take precautions to protect your hearing.

3. Obey safety regulations: Obey safety regulations and procedures to avoid head injuries and contact with ototoxic substances.

Tinnitus Prevention in the Home Environment

Tinnitus may be caused by several things in the home environment, such as loud noise exposure, head trauma, and ototoxic substances. Here are some ideas for making your house a safe place to live:

1. Reduce the volume: Dim the television, music, or other electrical gadgets.

2. Wear ear protection: If using power tools or other loud equipment is necessary, wear ear protection.

3. Avoid poisonous substances: Keep lead paint, insecticides, and other dangerous substances out of your home.

Tinnitus prevention via travel and leisure activities

Loud noise, head traumas, and ototoxic substances may all be encountered while traveling and in leisure activities. Following are some suggestions for avoiding tinnitus while traveling and having fun:

1. cover your ears: If you attend loud events like sports events or concerts, cover your ears.

2. Consider your exposure to noise whether wearing headphones, going to noisy events, or using equipment.

3. Obey safety rules: Obey safety rules while engaging in outdoor pursuits like skiing or snowboarding to avoid head injuries.

Tinnitus prevention may be greatly aided by modifications in the environment. Tinnitus may be avoided by reducing noise exposure, recognizing and avoiding job risks, making your home safe, and being aware of noise exposure when traveling and engaging in leisure activities. A person's chance of acquiring tinnitus may be decreased or its symptoms can be managed by implementing certain environmental adjustments.

Habits to Develop to Prevent Tinnitus

Certain practices may help prevent tinnitus, in addition to lifestyle adjustments and environmental alterations. We will go through some of the behaviors people may develop to prevent tinnitus, including using hearing protection, being aware of drugs that might result in tinnitus, consuming less alcohol, and quitting smoking.

Prevention of tinnitus and hearing protection

Tinnitus is often brought on by loud noise exposure, as we previously described. Wearing hearing protection is thus a crucial habit to develop to stop tinnitus. Following are a few applications for hearing protection:

1. Wear earplugs or earmuffs: When in loud places, such as at concerts or construction sites, wear earplugs or earmuffs.

Limit your exposure to loud noise by turning down the level on your electronic devices and staying away from noisy activities, for example.

3. Keep an eye on your hearing: Keep a frequent eye on it for any changes that could point to tinnitus or other hearing issues.

Preventing tinnitus with medication

As a side effect, several drugs might produce tinnitus. Therefore, another crucial habit to develop to avoid tinnitus is being aware of drugs and their possible negative effects. Managing drugs may be done in the following ways:

1. Consult your healthcare practitioner about any drugs you are now taking or intend to take to learn more about any possible adverse effects.

2. Follow dosage recommendations attentively and don't take more medication than is advised.

3 Report any adverse effects: If you notice any medication-related side effects, contact your doctor right away.

Prevention of Tinnitus and Alcohol

Tinnitus may also occur as a result of drinking alcohol. Therefore, cutting down on alcohol use is another crucial habit to develop to avoid tinnitus. Here are some suggestions for cutting less on drinking:

1. Set restrictions on the amount of alcohol you may drink each day or each week.

2. Steer clear of excessive drinking, which dramatically raises the risk of tinnitus.

3. Seek assistance: To cut down on drinking, ask for assistance from close friends, family members, or medical professionals.

Prevention of Tinnitus and Smoking

Tinnitus development is also more likely when smoking is present. So giving up cigarettes is another crucial habit to develop to prevent tinnitus. Here are some suggestions for quitting:

1. Seek support: If you want to stop smoking, ask your friends, family, or medical professionals for help.

2 Take into account nicotine replacement treatment: To lessen withdrawal symptoms, take into account employing nicotine replacement therapy, such as patches or gum.

3 Avoid triggers: Steer clear of things like stress and social settings that can make you want to smoke.

Tinnitus may be avoided by forming healthy habits including wearing hearing protection, being cautious while taking drugs, consuming less alcohol, and quitting smoking. These behaviors may help enhance general ear and hearing health and lessen the intensity of tinnitus symptoms.

CHAPTER THREE

Dealing with Tinnitus

Because tinnitus is a subjective condition that only the person experiencing it can notice, it may be difficult to control. There is presently no treatment for tinnitus, however, there are several management techniques that may help people deal with their symptoms. We will talk about coping mechanisms, sound treatment, tinnitus retraining therapy, counseling, and assistance for managing tinnitus.

Coping Techniques for Tinnitus Management

Individuals might use coping mechanisms to lessen the emotional and psychological effects of tinnitus. Here are a few coping mechanisms for dealing with tinnitus:

1. Mindfulness meditation: Practicing mindfulness meditation may help lessen tinnitus-related stress and anxiety.

2. Relaxation methods: Relaxation methods like progressive muscle relaxation, yoga, or deep breathing may help lower tension and anxiety.

3. Cognitive-behavioral treatment: People who have tinnitus may use this therapy to alter their unhelpful thinking and behavior patterns.

4. Distraction: You may reduce your tinnitus symptoms by taking part in fun activities like hobbies or listening to music.

Sound Therapy for Tinnitus Management

Tinnitus patients often get sound therapy, which uses sound to relieve symptoms.

Here are some alternatives for controlling tinnitus using sound therapy:

1. White noise is a continuous sound that may be used to hide the symptoms of tinnitus.

2. Music treatment: Music therapy entails listening to music that has been specially selected to address a person's unique tinnitus symptoms.

3. Sound machines: To assist conceal the symptoms of tinnitus, sound machines may provide a range of noises, such as rain or ocean waves.

Therapy for Tinnitus Retraining

The goal of tinnitus retraining treatment is to teach the brain to filter out tinnitus noises. Some elements of tinnitus retraining treatment include the following:

1. Sound treatment: Sound therapy, which may include the use of sound generators or hearing aids, is a crucial part of tinnitus retraining therapy.

2. Counseling: Counseling may assist people in developing coping mechanisms and a better understanding of their tinnitus.

3. Education: Learning more about tinnitus helps boost a person's attitude and lessen worry and tension.

Support and Counseling for Managing Tinnitus

Tinnitus sufferers must get counseling and assistance. Through counseling, people may learn coping mechanisms, have a greater understanding of their situation, and experience less stress and worry. Here are some resources for help and counseling in controlling tinnitus:

1. Support groups: Support groups may connect people with tinnitus to a community of others who share their struggles.

2. Individual therapy: Individual counseling may assist clients in coping mechanisms development and anxiety and tension reduction.

3. Family treatment: Through family therapy, tinnitus sufferers and their families may better comprehend the disease and learn coping mechanisms.

Tinnitus management is difficult, but several approaches and treatments may be used to assist people to manage their symptoms. Tinnitus sufferers may find that coping mechanisms, sound treatment, tinnitus retraining therapy, counseling, and support are all good management techniques. It's crucial to collaborate with a healthcare professional to create a personalized treatment plan that is appropriate for you.

Seeking Professional Tinnitus Help

Many people may seek professional assistance for their symptoms since tinnitus is a prevalent ailment that may be difficult to manage.

How and When to Get Tinnitus Medical Care

If you encounter any of the following symptoms in addition to tinnitus, it is essential to contact a doctor right away:

1. Sudden, acute, or recurrent tinnitus.

2. Tinnitus coupled with hearing loss, unsteadiness, or vertigo.

3. Tinnitus that is impairing your quality of life, for as by disrupting your sleep or impairing your focus.

4. Tinnitus that affects just one ear.

Types of Tinnitus Medical Treatments

Depending on the underlying cause of tinnitus, there are several medical therapies available. The following are a few tinnitus medical treatments:

1. Drugs: Tinnitus may be treated with drugs such as tricyclic antidepressants, benzodiazepines, or anticonvulsants.

2. Cognitive-behavioral treatment: People who are suffering from tinnitus may benefit from cognitive-behavioral therapy

to alter their unfavorable thinking and behavior patterns.

3. Tinnitus retraining therapy: This treatment may assist sufferers in rewiring their brains to block out tinnitus noises.

4. Hearing aids: People with hearing loss and tinnitus might benefit from hearing aids.

5. Tinnitus maskers: These tools create a sound to cover tinnitus noises.

Tinnitus Alternative Therapies

Medical tinnitus treatments may be combined with alternative remedies. Here are a few complementary treatments for tinnitus:

1. Acupuncture: Acupuncture is a treatment that includes inserting very thin needles into particular body sites to treat tinnitus symptoms.

2. Hypnotherapy: People who have tinnitus may relax and relieve tension and anxiety related to their symptoms with the aid of hypnotherapy.

3. Herbal treatments: Ginkgo biloba and zinc are two herbs that may help with tinnitus symptoms.

Guidelines for Interacting with Healthcare Professionals

Tinnitus patients who collaborate with medical professionals may create a successful treatment strategy. Here are some pointers for interacting with medical professionals:

1. Be honest and upfront: It's critical to tell your medical team the truth about your

symptoms and how they're impacting your life.

2. Ask questions: By inquiring, you may learn more about your disease and the suggested remedies.

3. Have patience: To create a successful treatment plan, it's crucial to have patience and work together with your doctor. Tinnitus control might take time.

In conclusion, those who have symptoms of tinnitus may find it helpful to seek expert assistance. Working with medical professionals, using complementary therapies, and receiving medical therapy may all help manage tinnitus symptoms. If you have frequent or severe tinnitus or if your symptoms are impairing your quality of life, you must contact a doctor. Working together with medical professionals may assist patients in creating a personalized treatment plan to control their tinnitus symptoms.

www.ingramcontent.com/pod-product-compliance
Lightning Source LLC
Chambersburg PA
CBHW051855250726
48659CB00006B/2221